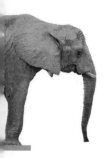

Mnemonics
for Surgery

Manoj Ramachandran BSc(Hons) MBBS(Hons)
MRCS(Eng) FRCS(Tr&Orth)
Paediatric and Young Adult Orthopaedic Fellow,
Royal National Orthopaedic Hospital Rotation,
Stanmore, Middlesex

Aaron Trinidade MBBS MRCS(Ed)
Senior House Officer in Otolaryngology,
Whipps Cross University Hospital, London

D1354090

PasTest
Dedicated to your success

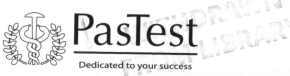

© 2006 PASTEST LTD
Egerton Court
Parkgate Estate
Knutsford
Cheshire
WA16 8DX

Telephone: 01565 752000

First Published 2006

ISBN: 1 904627 897
ISBN: 978 1 904627 890

A catalogue record for this book is available from the British Library.

The information contained within this book was obtained by the author from reliable sources. However, while every effort has been made to ensure its accuracy, no responsibility for loss, damage or injury occasioned to any person acting or refraining from action as a result of information contained herein can be accepted by the publishers or author.

PasTest Revision Books and Intensive Courses

PasTest has been established in the field of postgraduate medical education since 1972, providing revision books and intensive study courses for doctors preparing for their professional examinations.

Books and courses are available for the following specialties:

MRCGP, MRCP Parts 1 and 2, MRCPCH Parts 1 and 2, MRCPsych, MRCS, MRCOG Parts 1 and 2, DRCOG, DCH, FRCA, PLAB Parts 1 and 2.

For further details contact:

PasTest, Freepost, Knutsford, Cheshire WA16 7BR

Tel: 01565 752000   **Fax: 01565 650264**
www.pastest.co.uk   **enquiries@pastest.co.uk**

Text typeset and designed by Type Study, Scarborough, North Yorkshire

Printed and bound in the UK by MPG Books Ltd., Bodmin, Cornwall

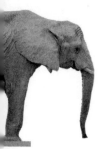

Mnemonic

1753, from the Greek *mnemonikos* 'of or pertaining to memory,' from *mnemon* (gen. *mnemonos*) 'remembering, mindful,' from *mnasthai* 'remember.'

Mnemosyne, lit. 'memory, remembrance,' was a Titaness, mother of the Muses.

Contents

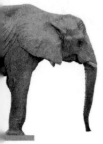

Acknowledgements	vi
Contributors	vii
Introduction	ix
Abbreviations	x
1. **Anatomy**	1
2. **Basic Sciences**	21
3. **General Topics**	29
4. **General Surgery, Vascular Surgery and Urology**	39
5. **Trauma**	51
6. **Orthopaedics**	59
7. **Miscellaneous**	81
Mnemonic Index	87
Subject Index	93

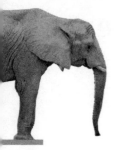

Acknowledgements

I would like to thank my wife Joanna for her support during all my projects. I must also give special mention to all those at PasTest for their continuing faith in my ideas.

Manoj Ramachandran

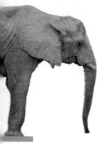

Contributors

Geoff Donald

David HA Jones

Harish Pai

Dishan Singh

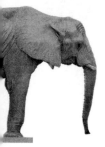

Introduction

Surgery is a rapidly evolving field and an ever-increasing amount of knowledge is expected of students and trainees both in the workplace and in professional examinations. Rapid recall of basic and advanced facts is therefore essential in such settings. Although individuals store and access information in multiple ways, there are recognised methods of learning and recall that can be utilised to make this process fun and efficient. One way that we have found to be very useful is by applying mnemonics to make mental associations between words and topics. Surely most of you, at one time or another, have used mnemonics in your learning? Remember GET SMASHED for the causes of acute pancreatitis or LOAF for the muscles of the hand supplied by the median nerve? If not, you'll find these mnemonics and many, many more in this book!

The aim of this book is to use mnemonics to cover the topics that are most often tested in surgery at all levels, from medical school to the final exit examination. Many or most (if not all) of these mnemonics have been begged, borrowed or stolen from a variety of sources (although we've put together quite a few of them from scratch). We sincerely apologise to those who we have stolen from without due credit. We take personal responsibility, so let us know and we will rectify the situation.

We hope you find this book both fun and informative, and that you will contribute to its contents in the future by supplying us with your own mnemonics (email them to mnemonicsfor surgery@pastest.co.uk).

Manoj Ramachandran & Aaron Trinidade

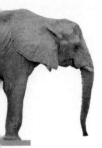

Abbreviations

AAA	Aortic abdominal aneurysm	DKA	Diabetic ketoacidosis
ACE	Angiotensin converting enzyme inhibitors	DVT	Deep vein thrombosis
		EBV	Epstein–Barr virus
		ERCP	Endoscopic retrograde cholangiopancreatography
AIDS	Acquired immune deficiency syndrome		
		FBC	Full blood count
ARDS	Acute respiratory distress syndrome	FRV	Functional residual capacity
AST	Aspartate aminotransferase	GA	General anaesthesia
		GCS	Glasgow Coma Score
CCF	Congestive cardiac failure	GI	Gastrointestinal
		Hb	Haemoglobin
CNS	Central nervous system	HIV	Human immunodeficiency virus
COPD	Chronic obstructive pulmonary disease		
		HRT	Hormone replacement therapy
CT	Computerised tomography	IBD	Inflammatory bowel disease
CTEV	Congenital talipes equinovarus		
		LDH	Lactate dehydrogenase
CVA	Cerebrovascular accident	MCPJ	Metacarpophalangeal joint
CVP	Central venous pressure	MEN	Multiple endocrine neoplasia
DDH	Developmental dysplasia of the hip	MOF	Multiple organ failure
		NBM	Nil by mouth
		NGT	Nasogastric tube
DEXA	Dual X-ray emission absorptiometry	NSAID	Nonsteroidal anti-inflammatory drugs
DIC	Disseminated intravascular coagulation		
		OCP	Oral contraceptive pill

PCA	Patient controlled analgesia	SCFE	Slipped capital femoral epiphysis
PE	Pulmonary embolism	TB	Tuberculosis
PEEP	Positive end-expiratory pressure	TIA	Transient ischaemic attack
PID	Pelvic inflammatory disease	TORCH	Toxoplasmosis, Rubella, Cytomegalovirus, Herpes
PIPJ	Proximal interphalangeal joint		
PTH	Parathyroid hormone	TPN	Total parenteral nutrition
PVNS	Pigmented villonodular synovitis	TSH	Thyroid stimulating hormone
SIRS	Systemic inflammatory response syndrome	UTI	Urinary tract infection
		WBC	White blood cell count

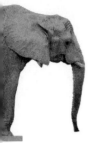

1. Anatomy

General

Derivatives of the branchial arches

Muscles **S**upport the **Pharynx** and **Larynx**

1st arch (**M**andibular arch; also known as **M**eckel's cartilage):
Muscles of **m**astication;
Mandible;
Mandibular nerve (cranial nerve V_3);
Mucous membrane (anterior two-thirds of tongue);
Maxillary artery

2nd arch (Hyoid arch):
Stapes;
Styloid process;
Stylohyoid ligament;
Superior part and lesser horn of hyoid bone;
Smiling muscles (of facial expression) and their nervous supply (CN VII)

3rd arch:
Stylo**pharyngeus** and glosso**pharyngeus** muscles;
Inferior part and greater horn of hyoid bone

4th and 6th arches:
The **larynx**:
Cartilages of the **larynx**: thyroid, cricoid, arytenoid, epiglottis;
Muscles of the **larynx**;
Pharyngeal and **laryngeal** parts of the vagus nerve (CN X)

5th arch: No derivatives

Potentially absent muscles

5 Ps

Palmaris longus
Plantaris
Peroneus tertius
Psoas minor
Pyramidalis

Remembering reflex roots

1,2 – buckle my shoe

3,4 – kick the door

5,6 – pick up sticks

7,8 – shut the gate

S**1,2** = ankle jerk
L**3,4** = knee jerk
C**5,6** = biceps and brachioradialis
C**7,8** = triceps

Important nerve supplies

C3, 4, 5 keep the diaphragm alive

(phrenic nerve)

C5, 6, 7 raise your arms to heaven

(long thoracic nerve of Bell to serratus anterior)

S 2, 3, 4 keep the erection, urine and faeces off the floor

(Sacral roots for erection, micturition and defecation)

Layers of the skin

Californians Love Girls in String Bikinis

Stratum **C**orneum
Stratum **L**ucidum
Stratum **G**ranulosum
Stratum **S**pinosum
Stratum **B**asale

Head and neck

Layers of the scalp

SCALP

Skin
sub**C**utaneous tissue
Aponeurosis and occipitofrontalis muscle
Loose subaponeurotic tissue
Pericranium

Nerve supply of the scalp

GLASS

Greater occipital / **G**reater auricular
Lesser occipital
Auriculotemporal
Supratrochlear
Supraorbital

Contents of the foramen ovale

OVALE

Otic ganglion (lies just inferior)
V$_3$ cranial nerve (mandibular part of trigeminal)
Accessory meningeal artery
Lesser petrosal nerve
Emissary veins

Structures passing through the supraorbital fissure

Luscious Fried Tomatoes Sit Naked In Anticipation Of Sauce

Lacrimal nerve
Frontal nerve
Trochlear nerve
Superior branch of oculomotor nerve
Nasociliary nerve
Inferior branch of oculomotor nerve
Abducent nerve
Ophthalmic veins
Sympathetic nerves

Nerve supply of the extraocular muscles

LR6, SO4 and the rest by 3

Lateral **R**ectus is supplied by the **6th** cranial nerve (abducens)
Superior **O**blique is supplied by the **4th** cranial nerve (trochlear)
Rest are all supplied by the **3rd** cranial nerve (oculomotor)

Cervical vertebral level landmarks

NoaH Told MariaH To Try Cervical Counting

C1: **N**ose (base), **H**ard palate
C2: **T**eeth
C3: **M**andible, **H**yoid bone
C4: **T**hyroid cartilage (upper)
C5: **T**hyroid cartilage (lower)
C6: **C**ricoid cartilage
C7: **C**ricoid cartilage (just below)

Muscle attachments to the hyoid bone

Colin, He Doesn't See Girls Much. That's Obvious, Stupid

Attaching superiorly:
Constrictor (middle)
Hyoglossus
Digastric
Stylohyoid
Geniohyoid
Myloyoid

Attaching inferiorly:
Thyrohyoid
Omohyoid
Sternohyoid

Branches of the superior thyroid artery

May I Slowly String Cat Gut?

Muscular
Infrahyoid
Superior laryngeal
Sternomastoid
Cricothyroid
Glandular

Branches of the external carotid artery

Some Anatomists Like Fishfingers, Others Prefer Sausage & Mash

Superior thyroid
Ascending pharyngeal
Lingual
Facial
Occipital
Posterior auricular
Superficial temporal
Maxillary

Tributaries of internal jugular vein

Medical Schools Let Confident People In

From inferior to superior:

Middle thyroid	**C**ommon facial
Superior thyroid	**P**haryngeal
Lingual	**I**nferior petrosal sinus

Upper limb

Innervation of serratus anterior

SALT

Serratus **A**nterior is supplied by the **L**ong **T**horacic nerve

$\left(c_{5-7} \right)$

Components of the brachial plexus

Robert Taylor Drinks Cold Beer

Roots $\left(C_{5-8} + {}^{T}1 \right)$

Trunks *superior, middle, inferior*

Divisions *(Ant. & Post × 3)*

Cords *lateral, medial, Posterior*

Branches

Remembering the brachial plexus

3:1:0:3:5:5

3 branches from roots (LSD)

Long thoracic nerve

Nerve to **S**ubclavius

Dorsal scapular nerve

1 from trunk

Suprascapular nerve

0 from divisions

3 branches from lateral cord (LML)

Lateral pectoral nerve
Musculocutaneous nerve
Lateral root of the median nerve

5 branches from medial cord (Miss Mary Makes Me Unhappy)

Medial pectoral nerve
Medial cutaneous nerve of forearm
Medial cutaneous nerve of arm
Medial root of median nerve
Ulnar nerve

5 branches from posterior cord (2 STAR)

2 Subscapular nerves (upper/lower)
Thoracodorsal nerve
Axillary nerve
Radial nerve

Innervation of the pectoralis muscles

Lateral is less, medial is more

Lateral pectoral nerves goes through pectoralis major
Medial pectoral nerves go through both pectoralis major and minor

Muscles of the rotator cuff

SITS

Suprapinatus
Infraspinatus
Teres minor
Subscapularis

Origins of the heads of the biceps muscle

Walk a SHORT way to the street CORner
Ride a LONG way on the SUPRAhighway

SHORT head of biceps originates from **COR**acoid process
of the scapula
LONG head originates from the **SUPRA**glenoid tubercle of
the scapula

Muscular attachments in and around the bicipital groove

A LaDy between two MAJORS

Pectoralis **major** attaches to lateral lip of bicipital groove
Teres **major** attaches to medial lip of bicipital groove
Latissimus **D**orsi attaches to the floor of bicipital groove in
between the two

Muscles supplied by the musculocutaneous nerve

BBC

Biceps
Brachialis
Coracobrachialis

Branches of the axillary artery

Send The Lord to Say A Prayer

From proximal to distal:
Superior thoracic
Thoracacromial
Lateral thoracic
Subscapular
Anterior circumflex humeral
Posterior circumflex humeral

Flexors of the elbow

Three Bs bend the elbow

Biceps
Brachialis
Brachioradialis

Some features of brachioradialis

BrachioRadialis

Beer-**R**aising muscle (flexes elbow with forearm in neutral)
Breaks the **R**ule in that it is a flexor **B**ut supplied by the **R**adial nerve
Behind it is the **R**adial nerve in the cubital fossa
Attaches to the **B**ottom of the **R**adius (distal aspect)

Contents of the cubital fossa

Really Need Booze To Be At My Nicest

From lateral to medial:
Radial **N**erve
Biceps **T**endon
Brachial **A**rtery
Median **N**erve

Appearance of elbow ossification centres by age

CRITOL

Site	Age
Capitellum	1–3
Radial head	3–5
Internal or medial epicondyle	5–7
Trochlea	7–9
Olecranon	9–11
Lateral epicondyle	11–13

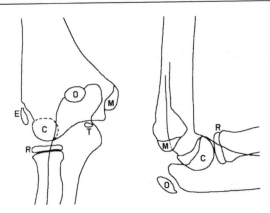

Forearm muscles: volar superficial group

Players Follow Pimps For Fun

Pronator teres
Flexor carpi radialis
Palmaris longus
Flexor carpi ulnaris
Flexor digitorum superficialis

Carpal bones

Some Lovers Try Positions

That They Cannot Handle

Proximal row   *Distal row*
Scaphoid   **T**rapezium
Lunate   **T**rapezoid
Triquetrum   **C**apitate
Pisiform   **H**amate
(Note that the trapezi**UM** is at the base of the th**UM**b)

Upper limb muscles supplied by the radial nerve

BREAST

Brachio**R**adialis
Extensors (forearm dorsal compartment)
Anconeus
Supinator
Triceps

Median and ulnar nerves

Some common features
Each supplies **1/2 of flexor digitorum profundus**
Each supplies **2 lumbricals**
Each has a **palmar cutaneous nerve**
Each supplies an **eminence group** of muscles (ulnar: hypothenar; median: thenar)
Each **enters forearm through two heads** (ulnar: heads of flexor carpi ulnaris; median: heads of pronator teres)
Each has **no branches in the upper arm**
Each makes **two fingers claw** when cut at the wrist
Each supplies a **palmaris** (median: palmaris longus; ulnar: palmaris brevis)

Hand muscles supplied by the median nerve

LOAF

Lateral two lumbricals   **A**bductor pollicis brevis
Opponens pollicis   **F**lexor pollicis brevis

Actions of the interossei muscles (supplied by the ulnar nerve)

PAD and DAB

Palmar interossei   **AD**duct
Dorsal interossei   **AB**duct

Intrinsic muscles of the hand

A OF A OF A

Thenar lateral to medial:
Abductor pollicis longus
Opponens pollicis
Flexor pollicis brevis
Adductor pollicis

Hypothenar lateral to medial:
Opponens digiti minimi
Flexor digiti minimi
Abductor digiti minimi

Trunk

Contents of the posterior mediastinum

3 GOOSE and 1 DUCK

Oesopha**GOOSE**
Azy**GOOSE** vein

Va**GOOSE** nerve
Thoracic **DUCK**

Contents of the superior mediastinum

PVT LEFT BATTLE

Phrenic nerve
Vagus nerve
Thoracic duct
LEFT recurrent laryngeal nerve (not the right)
Brachiocephalic veins
Aortic arch (and its 3 branches – see below)
Thymus
Trachea
Lymph nodes
o**E**sophagus

Branches of the aortic arch

The ABCS

Aortic arch gives off:
Brachiocephalic trunk
Left **C**ommon carotid artery
Left **S**ubclavian artery

Branches of descending abdominal aorta

Sometimes Intestines Get Really Stretched Causing Leakage

Suprarenals (paired)
Inferior mesenteric
Gonadal (paired)
Renals (paired)
Superior mesenteric
Coeliac
Lumbar (paired)

Tributaries of inferior vena cava

I Like To Rise So High

Iliacs
Lumbar
Testicular
Renal
Suprarenal
Hepatic vein

Retroperitoneal structures

SAD PUCKER

Suprarenal glands
Aorta and inferior vena cava
Duodenum (half)
Pancreas
Ureters
Colon (ascending and descending)
Kidneys
o**E**sophagus (anterior and left covered)
Rectum

Bronchopulmonary segments of the left lung

Astute Anatomists Share Inside Secrets About Lungs

Apicoposterior (S1&2)
Anterior (S3)
Superior (S4)
Inferior (S5)
Superior (S6)
Anteromedial basal (S7+8)
Lateral basal (S9)

Length of the parts of four parts of the duodenum

Count 1 to 4 but staggered

1st part	2 inches
2nd part	3 inches
3rd part	4 inches
4th part	1 inch

Apertures in the diaphragm

Come Enter the Abdomen

T8	inferior vena **C**ava (caval foramen)
T10	o**E**sophagus (oesophageal hiatus)
T12	**A**orta (aortic hiatus)

Each of the 3 holes have 3 structures passing through them

Caval foramen	Inferior vena cava, right phrenic nerve, lymph nodes
o**E**sophageal hiatus	Oesophagus, vagal trunks, left gastric vessels
Aortic hiatus	Aorta, thoracic duct, azygous vein

Important facts about the spleen

1,3,5,7,9,11

Dimensions **1** inch × **3** inches × **5** inches
Weight **7** ounces
Underlies ribs **9** to **11**

Branches of the lumbar plexus

I (twice) Get Lost On Fridays

Iliohypogastric (L1)
Ilioinguinal (L1)
Genitofemoral (L1, L2)
Lateral femoral cutaneous (L2, L3)
Obturator (L2, L3, L4)
Femoral (L2, L3, L4)

Zones of the adrenal cortex

GFR

Zona **G**lomerulosa
Zona **F**asciculata
Zona **R**eticularis

Remembering lumbar plexus roots

2 from 1, 2 from 2, 2 from 3

2 nerves from 1 root: ilioinguinal (L1), iliohypogastric (L1)
2 nerves from 2 roots: genitofemoral (L1,L2), lateral femoral (L2,L3)
2 nerves from 3 roots: obturator (L2,L3,L4), femoral (L2,L3,L4)

Autonomic supply to the penis

Point and Shoot

Parasympathetic **P**oints it up (erection)
Sympathetic **S**hoots it out (ejaculation)

Borders of the inguinal canal

Friendly Irish Anaesthetist Offers Ronaldo A Painless Tendon

Floor	**I**nguinal ligament
Anterior wall	**O**bliques (internal and external)
Roof	**A**rching fibres of tranversalis and internal oblique
Posterior wall	**T**ransversalis fascia

Contents of the spermatic cord

Piles Don't Contribute To A Good Sex Life

Pampiniform plexus
Ductus deferens
Cremasteric artery
Testicular artery
Artery of the ductus deferens
Genital branch of the genitofemoral nerve
Sympathetic nerve fibres
Lymphatic vessels

Order of structures within the femoral sheath

NAVEL

From lateral to medial (towards the navel!):
Nerve
Artery
Vein
Empty space
Lymph node (of Cloquet)

Boundaries of the femoral triangle

So I May Always Love Sally

Superiorly: **I**nguinal ligament
Medially: **A**dductor longus
Laterally: **S**artorius

Layers of the scrotum

Some Damn Englishman Called It The Testis

Skin
Dartos muscle
External spermatic fascia
Cremaster muscle
Internal spermatic fascia
Tunica vaginalis
Testis

Lower limb

External rotators of the femur

Pretty Girls Often Get Old Quickly

Piriformis
Gemellus superior
Obturator internus
Gemellus inferior
Obturator externus
Quadratus femoris

Medial compartment of the thigh

3 DUCks PECking On GRAss

adADUCtor longus → ad**DUC**tor longus
ad**DUC**tor longus
ad**DUC**tor brevis
ad**DUC**tor magnus
PECtineus
Obturator externus
GRAcilis

Branches of the superficial femoral artery

Put My Leg Down Please

Profunda femoris (deep femoral artery)
Medial circumflex femoral artery
Lateral circumflex femoral artery
Descending genicular arteries
Perforating arteries

Tendons of pes anserinus

Say Grace before Tea

Sartorius (supplied by femoral nerve)
Gracilis (supplied by obturator nerve)
Semi**T**endinosus (supplied by tibial division of sciatic nerve)

Tarsal bones

Curtis Can't Count Bones, Never Took Calculus

Cuneiform (medial)
Cuneiform (intermediate)
Cuneiform (lateral)
cu**B**oid
Navicular
Talus
Calcaneum

Eversion versus inversion of the ankle

The second letter rule

Evertors:
pErineus longus
pErineus brevis
pErineus tertius

Invertors:
tIbialis posterior
tIbialis anterior

Structures passing behind the medial malleolus

Tom, Dick and A Very Nervous Harry

Tibialis posterior
flexor Digitorum longus
posterior tibial Artery
posterior tibial Vein
posterior tibial Nerve
flexor Hallucis longus

Structures passing in front of the ankle (from medial to lateral)

Tom Has A Very Nasty Dirty Pill

Tibialis anterior
extensor Hallucis longus
dorsalis pedis Artery
anterior tibial Vein
deep peroneal Nerve
extensor Digitorum
Peroneus tertius

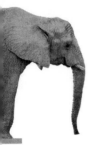

2. Basic sciences

Everything you need to know about collagen

COLLAGEN

C-terminal propeptide (procollagen)/**C**ovalent **C**rosslinks/ **C**onnective tissue such as **C**artilage/contains **C**hondroblasts/**C**opper **C**ofactor in formation
Outside the cell is where collagen normally functions/ **O**steogenesis imperfecta
Long triple helical fibres
Ligaments
Alpha chains/**A**ttached by H bonds form triple helix
Glycine in every third position/**GO**lgi allows procollagen to **GO** outside of cell
Extracellular matrix/**E**yes (cornea, sclera)/**E**hlers–Danlos syndrome
N-terminal propeptide (procollagen)/**N**onhelical terminal extensions
Note: Procollagen **LEAVE**s the cell to be c**LEAVE**d by procollagen peptidases

Facts about cartilage

The As

Aneural
Avascular
Alymphatic
Anaerobic
Anisotropic
Aggrecan is a major proteoglycan

Causes of high potassium

HI POTASSIuM

Hypoaldosteronism (Addison's disease)
Iatrogenic (excess infusion)
Potassium-sparing diuretics (eg spironolactone)
Oliguria
Tissue destruction (rhabdomyolysis, burns)
Acidosis
Spurious (lab error; very common!)
Suxamethonium (inducing agent in anaesthesia)
Ingestion (potassium iodide, bananas, citrus)
Massive blood transfusion

Causes of low potassium

CRAMPING

Cushing's/**C**onn's syndromes
Renal tubular failure
Alkalosis
Mucus per rectum (villous adenoma; important surgical cause!)
Pyloric stenosis
Intestinal fistulae
Nasogastric aspiration
GI upset (vomiting and diarrhoea)

Causes of high sodium

SALTED

Sweating
Addison's disease
Lack of fluids (common cause on the wards!)
TPN
Emesis (vomiting)
Diabetes insipidus/**D**ehydration

Causes of hypercalcaemia

HI CALCIUM Produces Stones

Hyperparathyroidism(primary, secondary or tertiary)/**H**ypocalcuric hypercalcaemia (familial)
Iatrogenic: thiazide diuretics
Calcium and vitamins A and D excess
Addison's disease/**A**cromegaly
Lung (pulmonary) tuberculosis
Carcinoma (breast, prostate, lung, kidney, thyroid)
Immobility
Unrelated: ectopic PTH production (lung, kidney, ovary carcinoma)
Multiple myeloma/**M**ilk-alkali syndrome (rare)
Paget's disease of bone
Sarcoidosis ($\uparrow$ vitamin D action)

Symptoms of hypercalcaemia

Bones, stones, moans and psychic groans

Bones: Excessive bone resorption
Stones (renal): Polyuria, polydipsia, dehydration and kidney stones
Moans (gastrointestinal): Constipation, peptic ulcer disease and pancreatitis
Psychic groans (CNS): Confusion and stupor

Virchow's triad of risk factors for venous thrombosis

VIRchow

Vascular trauma
Increased coagulability
Reduced blood flow (stasis)

Possible fates of a thrombus

DOPE

Dissolution
Organisation and repair
Propagation
Embolisation

Vitamin-K-dependent factors that are inactivated by warfarin

Some Tend To Nicely Stop Clots

Seven
Ten
Two
Nine
Protein S
Protein C

Causes of avascular necrosis

PLASTIC RAG

Pancreatitis
Perthes' disease
Lupus
Alcohol*
Atherosclerosis
Steroids*
Sickle cell disease
Trauma

Idiopathic*
Caisson's disease
Radiation
Amyloidosis
Gaucher's disease
*most common

Side-effects of corticosteroids
I WAS HOPPING MAD

Infection
Wasting
Adrenal insufficiency
Sugar disturbances (diabetes)
Hypotension
Osteoporosis
Peptic ulcer
Pancreatitis
Proximal myopathy
Incidental (moon facies, hirsutism)
Necrosis of the femoral head
Glaucoma/cataracts
MAD (psychological changes)

Adverse effects on wound healing
VITAMINS A, B, C, D, E

Vitamin deficiency
Infection (local and general)
Technique
Arterial supply (especially vascular disease or trauma)
Malnutrition
Icterus (secondary to hepatobiliary disease, haemolysis or uraemia)
Necrotic tissue
Sugar (diabetes mellitus)
Anaemia/Age
Blood clot (haematoma formation)

Cancer (local or distant)
Drugs (cytotoxic agents and steroids)
Edge tension (especially in obesity)

Types of hypersensitivity reaction

ACIDE

I	Anaphylactic
II	Cytotoxic-mediated
III	Immune complex
IV	Delayed hypersensitivity
V	Excitatory antibodies*

* Seen in Graves' disease

Causes of acquired immunodeficiency

Immunodeficiency May Directly Cause Life-threatening Sepsis

Infections (EBV, parvovirus, malaria, HIV)
Malignancy (leukaemia, lymphoma)
Drugs (azathioprine, steroids, radiotherapy)
Chronic renal failure (combined B- and T-cell deficiencies)
Loss of individual components of the immune system (as in nephrotic syndrome)
Splenectomy

Differences between apoptosis and necrosis

LIFELESS

	Apoptosis	Necrosis
Leaky membranes	✓	✓
Inflammatory response	✗	✓
Fate	Swallowed by neighbouring cells	Phagocytosed by macrophages
Extent	Confined to single cell	Groups of cells involved
Laddering*	✗	✓
Energy dependent	✗	✓
Swell or shrink	Shrink	Swell
Stimulus	Physiological or pathological	Pathological only

*Laddering: hallmark pattern seen on gel electrophoresis caused by fragmented DNA

Three types of muscle

Muscle Contraction Results Mainly Through Sustained Action Potentials

	Skeletal	Cardiac	Smooth
Motor end plates	✓	✗	✗
Cytology	Cylindrical fibres	Branched fibres	Fusiform fibres
Response	Graded	All or nothing	Graded
Mitochondria	Few	Many	Few
Tetany	✓	✗	✓
Sarcomeres	✓	✓	✗
ATPase	✓✓✓	✓✓	✓
Pacemaker	✗	✓	✓(slow)

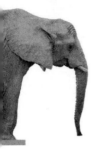

3. General topics

Basics of diagnosis

Describing any disease

Dressed In A Surgeon's Gown, A Physician May Make Some Initial Temporary Progress

Definition
Incidence
Age
Sex
Geography
Aetiology
Pathology
Macropathology
Micropathology
Signs/**S**ymptoms
Investigations
Treatment
Prognosis

Taking a pain history

SOCRATES

Site
Onset
Character
Radiation/**R**elieving factors
Associated factors
Treatment
Exacerbating factors
Severity

Taking a social history

CHAPTER

Company, eg friends, neighbours, family
Housing, eg stairs, heating, telephone
Activities, eg washing, dressing, cooking
Pleasure, eg smoking, sex, hobbies, alcohol
Travel, eg national, international
Employment, eg temporary, permanent
Requirements, eg home help, social worker

Examining lumps

Should The Children Ever Find Lumps Readily

Site/**S**ize/**S**hape/**S**urface/**S**ymmetry/**S**kin changes
Temperature/**T**enderness/**T**ransilluminability/**T**ransmitted
pulsations/**T**ethering to overlying structures
Consistency (soft, firm, or hard)/**C**olour
Edge/**E**xpansility
Fluid thrill/**F**ixed (or mobile)
Lumps elsewhere/**L**ymph nodes
Resonance

Examining ulcers

BEDS

Base
Edge
Depth/**D**ischarge
Size/**S**ite/**S**hape/**S**urrounding tissues

Reading any X-ray

ABCs

Appropriateness (right patient?)/**A**dequacy (eg penetration, all areas visualised)/**A**lignment
Bones
Cartilage
Soft tissues

Differential diagnosis of any condition

TIN CAN BED

Trauma
Infection/**I**nflammation/**I**diopathic/**I**atrogenic
Neoplastic
Congenital
Arteriovenous
Nutritional
Biochemical
Endocrine
Degenerative/**D**rug-induced

Perioperative issues

Obtaining consent for an operation

PRO AND CON

Procedure and **P**rognosis
Risks
Other information, eg drains, blood transfusion
Alternatives, eg non-surgical options
No force applied to the patient
Demonstration of understanding by patient
CONdition explained adequately

Common postoperative complications

(Consent every patient for these complications)

SHIP

Scar
Haematoma
Infection
Pain

Causes of postoperative pyrexia

The 8 Cs

Catheter (urinary tract infection)
Cannula/**C**entral line (phlebitis or drug allergy)
Cut/**C**ellulitis
Chest (atelectasis or PE)
Calf (DVT days 7–10)
Collection (of pus, eg pelvic, subphrenic)

Causes of pulmonary embolism
TOM SCHREPFER

Trauma
Obesity
Malignancy (hypercoagulable state)
Surgery (especially orthopaedic and pelvic)
Cardiac disease
Hospitalisation (prolonged)
Rest (bed-ridden patients)
Elderly
Past history of DVT/PE/pregnancy
Fracture (especially of long bones)
o**E**strogen (OCP, HRT)
Road trip (eg long flight)

Causes of postoperative confusion
DELIRIUM

Drugs
Electrolyte imbalance
Lack of drugs (alcohol/heroin withdrawal)
Infection (sepsis)
Reduced sensory input (new surroundings, blindness)
Intracranial problems (TIA, stroke, post-ictal state)
Urinary retention
Myocardial problems (infarction, arrhythmias)

Anaesthesia and intensive care

Aims of surgical anaesthesia
The 5 As

Anaesthesia
Analgesia
Areflexia
Amnesia
Autonomic stability

Types of drugs used as premedication

The 6 As

Anxiolytics: commonly benzodiazapines
Amnesics
Analgesics
Antacids: reduce gastric acid load
Anti-autonomics: to prevent vagally mediated bradycardia and to reduce secretions
Antiemetics: commonly dopamine or histamine antagonists

Indications for transfer to surgical intensive care

Only Real Frail Admissions Require Care

One-to-one nursing
Renal replacement therapy
Fluid and electrolyte abnormalities
Airway support (with or without ventilation)
Respiratory failure requiring ventilation
Cardiovascular monitoring

Types and causes of hypoxia

HASH

(smoking hash causes hypoxia!)

Hypoxic hypoxia:	Airway problem; shunt present; low inspired O_2
Anaemic hypoxia:	Hb low or abnormal; carboxyHb; metHb
Stagnant hypoxia:	(also known as ischaemic hypoxia) ↑afterload, ↓preload, ↓contractility
Histotoxic hypoxia:	Cyanide poisoning

Patients at risk of hypoxia

SCOPE

Smokers/**S**urgery (abdominal, orthopaedic)
COPD
Obesity ($\downarrow$ FRC)
Preoperative opiates
Elderly ($\downarrow$ FRC)

Indications for intubation and mechanical ventilation

3As and 4Hs

Airway protection: GCS < 8
Airway toilet and secretion control
Apnoeic patient
Head injury for control of P_aCO_2 (aiming for normocapnoea)
Hypoxaemia P_aO_2 < 8 kPa
Hypoventilation with hypercapnoea and acidosis
Hyperventilation (respiratory rate > 35 breaths per minute)
with impending exhaustion

Indications for tracheostomy

CRIMP PRINTS

Congenital (laryngeal webs, subglottic stenosis)
Radiotherapy (to neck causing stenosis)
Infections (epiglottis, Ludwig's angina)
Malignancy
Protection of bronchotracheal tree
Paralysis (bilateral) of cords
Respiratory failure
Intubation (prolonged)
Neurological (eg myasthenia gravis, multiple sclerosis)
Trauma to upper airway
Secretions (bronchial)

Causes of ARDS

BEAT ARDS

Blood transfusion (massive)/**B**urns
Embolism (fat, air or amniotic fluid)
Aspiration
Trauma (polytrauma, direct chest trauma)
Acute pancreatitis
Radiation (eg post-radiotherapy)
DIC/**D**rug overdose/near-**D**rowning/**D**ialysis/**D**iffuse
pneumonia (viral, fungal or bacterial)
Sepsis/**S**hock/**S**moke inhalation

Management of ARDS

ARDS

Avoid causes of pulmonary oedema (eg CCF, pneumonia)
Respiratory assistance (mechanical ventilation, eg PEEP)
Dependent body positions (gravity ↑ lung blood flow)
Secretions (avoid with help of physiotherapist)

Indications for central line insertion

CHIPS

CVP monitoring/**C**ardiac pacing
Haemodialysis
Infusions (TPN, chemotherapy)
Pulmonary artery catheterisation
Shoddy peripheral venous access

Patients at risk of renal failure

LORD help these patients!

Liver disease (especially obstructive jaundice)
Obstructive nephropathy (ie post-renal failure secondary to
urinary retention, eg post-prostatectomy clot, UTI)/**O**ld
people

Renal vascular disease (diabetic nephropathy, atherosclerotic renal disease)
Drugs (NSAIDs, ACE inhibitors)

Renal causes of renal failure

CHIMP

Contrast media
Haemodialysis products (Hb, urea)
Immunoglycosides (eg gentamicin)
Myoglobinuria (crush injuries)
Poor perfusion (acute tubular necrosis)

Indications for renal dialysis

AEIOU

Acid–base problems (severe alkalosis/acidosis)
Electrolyte problems (hyperkalaemia)
Intoxication (eg antifreeze)
Overload (fluid)
Uraemia (symptomatic)

Epidemiology

Types of study designs

ECCCI

Ecological (done at population level on basis of place and time)
Cross-sectional (measures prevalence at any point in time)
Case–control (the study of rare diseases)
Cohort [either the study of specific conditions or exposure over a period of time (temporal sequence) or the study of rare risk factors]
Interventional (clinical trials: measures effectiveness of intervention and tests causal hypotheses)

Criteria for a screening programme

IATROGENIC

Important health problem with its **I**ncidence known
Accepted and effective treatment available
Treatment and diagnostic facilities available
Recognisable latent and early symptomatic stage or stages present
Opinions on who to treat agreed
Guaranteed safety, sensitivity and specificity of the test
Examination and/or treatment are acceptable to the patient.
Natural history of the condition known
Inexpensive and simple tests
Cost-effective screening program which is **C**ontinuously rolled out and repeated at intervals

Problems associated with screening

D SCUM

Delay in receiving results/**D**istress of patient on learning further assessment is needed
Sensitivity/**S**pecificity
Cost
Uptake
Methodology

Components of the audit cycle

As Shops Opened, Colin Invested Excitedly

Agree on an **A**im
Set **S**tandards
Observe clinical practice
Compare practice with standards
Implement change
Evaluate change

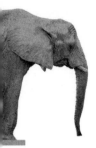

4. General surgery, vascular surgery and urology

Abdominal wall, upper gastro-intestinal and biliary tract

Umbilical hernia in children

The rule of 3s

3% of live births
3:1000 need repair
Repair done only after **age 3**
Recur in **3rd trimester** of pregnancy

Risk factors for oesophageal carcinoma

ABCDEF

Achalasia
Barrett's oesophagus
Corrosives
Diet
o**E**sophageal webs
Familial

Indications for surgery in peptic ulcer disease

I CHOP

Intractability (failed medical management)
Cancer (gastric ulcers only)
Haemorrhage
Obstruction (gastric outlet obstruction secondary to scarring/stricture formation)
Perforation

Risk factors for gallstones

The 6Fs

Fat
Female
Fair
Fertile
Flatulent
Forty-plus

Causes of hepatomegaly

CHARM TIPS

Cirrhosis / CCF
Haematological, eg lymphoma
Amyloid
Reye's syndrome/Riedel's lobe
Metabolic, eg Gaucher's disease
Tumour (primary and secondary)
Infection (viral, bacterial and protozoal)
Portal hypertension/Polycystic disease
Sarcoidosis

Causes of splenomegaly

CHIASMA

Congestion, eg portal hypertension
Haematological, eg lymphoma
Infarction, eg post-bacterial endocarditis
Acquired infections (eg viral, bacterial)
Storage diseases, eg Gaucher's disease
Masses, eg cysts
Autoimmune, eg Felty's syndrome in rheumatoid arthritis

Pancreas

Causes of acute pancreatitis

GET SMASHED

Gallstones (leading cause in UK)
Ethanol
Trauma
Steroids
Mumps (also Coxsackie)
Autoimmune (polyarteritis nodosa)
Scorpion bite (common in Trinidad)
Hypercalcaemia/**H**ypothermia/**H**yperlipidaemia
ERCP/**E**mboli
Drugs (thiazides, azathioprine, oestrogens)

Prognosis of pancreatitis (Ranson's criteria)

GA LAW and COUCH

At presentation:
Glucose >10 mmol/l (patient not diabetic)
Age >55 years (or >70 if gallstones)
LDH >350 iu/l
AST > 250 iu/l
WBC >16,000·10^9/l

During the next 48 hours:
Calcium <2.0 mmol/l (corrected)
Oxygen (*P*O$_2$) <8 kPa or 60 mmHg
Urea increase >10 mmol/l despite IV fluids
Concealed (ie estimated sequestered) fluid >6 l
Haematocrit increase >10%
1 point is given for each criterion present, severe
pancreatitis = 3 or more points

Causes of raised amylase

AMYLASE

AAA rupture/**A**cidosis (diabetic ketoacidosis)
Mesenteric ischaemia
g**Y**naecological pathology (ovarian tumour)
Liver disease
Anuria (renal failure)
Salivary gland disease (tumour, inflammation)/**S**tomach
ulcer (perforated)
Ectopic pregnancy

Treatment of pancreatitis

PANCREAS

Proton pump inhibitors
Analgesia (PCA)
NBM
Catheterise
Rehydrate (IV fluids)
Empty stomach (NGT)
Antibiotics (severe only)
Sliding scale insulin (if blood sugar high)

Complications of pancreatitis

PANCREAS

Pseudocyst/**P**hlegmon
Airway problems (ARDS, pleural effusion)/**A**scites/**A**bscess
Necrosis (may lead to haemorrhagic pancreatitis)

Coagulation disorder, eg DIC/calcium deficit
Renal failure
Encephalopathy
Arterial (splenic/mesenteric/portal vessel rupture or
thrombosis)
Sugar (diabetes)/SIRS/Sepsis

Lower gastrointestinal

Causes of right iliac fossa pain

APPENDICITIS

Appendicitis/Abscess
PID/Period pains
Pancreatitis
Ectopic pregnancy/Endometriosis
Neoplasia
Diverticulitis
Intussusception
Crohn's disease/Cyst (ovarian)
IBD
Torsion (ovary)
Irritable bowel syndrome
Stones (urolithiasis)

Complications of appendicitis

WRAP IF HOT

Wound infection
Respiratory problems (atelectasis, pneumonia)
Abscess (pelvic)
Portal pyaemia
Ileus (paralytic)
Faecal fistula
Hernia (right inguinal)
Obstruction (adhesions)
Thromboembolic phenomenon (DVT/PE)

Meckel's diverticulum

The rule of 2s

Occurs in **2**% of the population
2:1 male:female ratio
Approximately **2** inches long
Found **2** feet from the ileocaecal junction
1 in 2 will contain ectopic tissue (gastric or pancreatic)
Only **2**% are symptomatic
Important cause of rectal bleeding in **under 2**s

Indications for stoma formation

FLEDD

Feeding: gastrostomy, jejunostomy (eg post GI surgery or in CNS disease)
Lavage: caecostomy (eg on-table bowel prep before distal colonic surgery; used rarely)
Exteriorisation: colostomy, ileostomy
Decompression: caecostomy (in gross bowel obstruction; rarely used now)
Diversion: ileostomy, colostomy, duodenostomy (following duodenal trauma; rare)

Complications of stomas

STOMA BAGS HELP

*S*tenosis
*T*ight defect (narrow abdominal wall defect leading to **ischaemia/gangrene**)
Overflow (of afferent bowel contents into efferent limb; may compromise distal anastomosis)
Maintenance problems (stoma nurse/education helps)
Anaemia (especially megaloblastic due to terminal ileal loss in ileostomy)
Bloating (flatus may be a problem)
Aroma (malodour; helped with deodorants)

Gallbladder/kidney stones (due to loss of terminal ileum/bile salt absorption; and dehydration respectively)
Short-gut syndrome (excess fluid/electrolyte loss)
Hernia *(parastomal)*
Excoriation *(of skin, especially in ileostomy)*
Leakage *(usually secondary to ill-fitting device)*
Prolapse *(may need re-fashioning)*
(Not listed in order of importance. Complications in italics are primary)

Conditions preventing closure of fistulae
FRIEND

Foreign body
Radiation
Infection
Epithelialisation
Neoplasia
Distal obstruction

Causes of functional obstruction
CRAMPED

CVA (stroke)
Renal failure
Retroperitoneal haemorrhage
Abdominal malignancy
MI/**M**yxoedema/**M**esenteric vascular disease
Post-operative/**P**neumonia/**P**eritonitis/**P**elvic abscess
Electrolyte disturbance
Damaged bones (eg orthopaedic trauma)
Drugs (tricyclic antidepressants, GA)/**D**iabetic ketoacidosis

Features of Gardner's syndrome

GARDENS

GI tumours eg colonic adenomatous polyps
Abnormal dentition
Ribs and other bony abnormalities, eg exostoses
Desmoid tumours
Endocrine tumours, eg thyroid carcinoma
Nervous system tumours, eg medulloblastoma
Soft tissue tumours, eg epidermoid (sebaceous) cysts

Vascular surgery

Symptoms and signs of acute limb ischaemia

The 6 Ps

Pain
Pallor
Paraesthesia
Paralysis
Pulselessness
Poikilothermia (perishing with cold)

Causes of aneurysms

Aneurysms May Sometimes Cause Terrible Bleeding

Atherosclerosis (most common cause)
Mycotic (secondary to endocarditis)
Syphilitic
Connective tissue disorders, eg Marfan's syndrome,
Ehlers-Danlos syndrome
Trauma
Berry aneurysm (and other congenital aneurysms)

Indications for amputation

The 3 Ds

Dead limb (eg peripheral vascular disease causing critical ischaemia/gangrene; most common reason in UK)
Dead loss (eg trauma, neurological disease)
Deadly (eg osteosarcoma, septic limb)

Complications of varicose veins

AEIOU

Aching
Eczema
Itching
Oedema
Ugly (lipodermatosclerosis, haemosiderin deposition, varicosities)

Signs of chronic venous insufficiency

HEAVE

Haemosiderin deposition (secondary to blood stasis)
Eczema (venous)
Ankle ulcers (over medial gaiter region)
Varicose veins
o**E**dema

Order of skin changes in Raynaud's phenomenon

WBC

White
Blue
Crimson (red)

Causes of secondary Raynaud's

BAD CaT

Blood disorders, eg polycythaemia
Arterial, eg atherosclerosis, Buerger's disease
Drugs, eg beta blockers, oral contraceptive pill
Connective tissues disorders, eg rheumatoid arthritis, systemic lupus erythematosus, scleroderma, polyarteritis nodosa
Trauma, eg vibration injury

Urology

Differential diagnosis of haematuria

HEMATURIA

Hereditary (eg Osler–Weber–Rendu syndrome)/Henoch Schonlein purpura
Embolism (infective endocarditis)
Malignant hypertension
Acute and chronic glomerulonephritis/Ig**A** nephropathy
Tumours/**T**rauma/**T**oxic drugs
Urolithiasis
Renal papillary necrosis
Infection (pyelonephritis, cystitis, urethritis, tuberculosis)
Anticoagulants

Differential diagnosis of scrotal swellings

THE THEATRES

Torsion
Hernia
Epididymitis
Trauma
Hydrocoele (and varicocoele)
o**E**dema
Appendix of the testis (torsion)

Tumour/Tuberculosis
Recurrent leukaemia
Epididymal cyst
Syphilis

Complications of undescended testis

TESTIS

Trauma
Epididymo-orchitis
Sterility
Torsion
Interstitial hernia
Seminoma

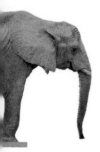

5. Trauma

Management of soft tissue injuries

PRICE

Painkillers
Rest
Ice
Compression
Elevation

Advanced Trauma Life Support (ATLS)

ABCDE

Airway with cervical spine control
Breathing
Circulation with haemorrhage control
Disability
Exposure

Disability assessment in ATLS

AVPU

Alert
Responds to **V**ocal stimuli
Responds to **P**ainful stimuli
Unresponsive

Glasgow coma score

VEM

Verbal (out of 5 – see OCAIN below)
Eye (out of 4 – use AVPU as above)
Motor (out of 6)

Glasgow coma score (verbal)

Like taking more and more cOCAINe

Oriented
Confused
in**A**ppropriate
Incomprehensible
None

Life-threatening conditions in the ATLS primary survey

ATOMIC

Airway obstruction
Tension pneumothorax
Open pneumothorax
Massive haemothorax
Incipient flail chest
Cardiac tamponade

Features of pneumothorax

P-THORAX

Pleuritic pain
Tracheal deviation
Hyper-resonance
Onset sudden
Reduced breath sounds
Absent fremitus
X-ray shows collapse

A quick history for trauma

AMPLE

Allergies
Medications
Past medical history
Last meal
Event itself

Considerations in a road traffic accident

I AM SCARED

Impact (eg head-on, rear-end)
Automobile versus pedestrian, push bike or motorcycle
Medical history
Speed
Compartment intrusion
Age
Restraints (lap and shoulder, airbag, infant or child seat)
Ejection/**E**xtrication
Death (eg at scene, within same vehicle)

Classes of haemorrhage in trauma

Like a game of tennis (Love-15-30-40)

0–15	<15%	Up to 750 ml loss
15–30	15–30%	800–1500 ml loss
30–40	30–40%	1500–2000 ml loss
Game over	>40%	>2000 ml loss

Seven types of bone fractures

As heard on Star Wars, GO C3PO

Greenstick
Open
Complete
Closed
Comminuted
Pathological
Others, eg growth plate injuries

Gustillo–Anderson classification of open fractures

Grade I to III then ABC

Grade I	Minimally contaminated wound less than 1 cm long
Grade II	Moderately contaminated wound more than 1 cm long
Grade III	Highly contaminated wound with extensive soft tissue damage
A	**A**dequate soft tissue cover
B	**B**one exposed
C	**C**irculatory compromise requiring repair

Common dislocations

The 90% rule

>90% of shoulder dislocations are anterior
>90% of hip dislocations are posterior

Compartment syndrome

All the Ps

Early
Pain out of proportion to the injury
Pain with passive motion

Later
Paralysis
Pulselessness
Paraesthesia
Pallor
Poikilothermia (or **P**erishing with cold)

Causes of delayed or non union
SPLINT

Soft tissue interposition
Position of reduction, eg gapping
Loss of blood supply/**L**oss of bone
Infection
Nutrition (mal)
Tumours and other pathological conditions

Reducing an anteriorly dislocated shoulder (Kocher's manoeuvre)
TEAM

Traction
External rotation
Adduction
Medial rotation

Causes of posterior shoulder dislocation (other than trauma)
The 3 Es

Epileptic seizure
Electric shock
Electroconvulsive therapy

Monteggia and Galeazzi fractures

3 types of MURG

First: **M**onteggia = **U**lna fracture with **R**adial head **G**one (dislocated)
Second: **M**onteggia = **U**lna fracture, **R**adial fracture = **G**aleazzi
Third: **M**onteggia occurs **U**p near the elbow; it's the **R**everse for **G**aleazzi (down near the wrist)

Management of intracapsular neck of femur fractures

1, 2 – Try to screw

3, 4 – Austin Moore

Based on Garden's classification, for lower grades (1, 2), a head-preserving procedure (try to screw) is attempted, such as cannulated screw fixation, while for higher grades (3, 4), the head is removed and a hemiarthroplasty (eg an Austin Moore prosthesis) is performed.

Salter–Harris classification of fractures around the physis

SALTR

I – **S**eparation
II – **A**bove (through metaphysis)
III – **L**ower than (through epiphysis)
IV – **T**hrough (metaphysis and epiphysis)
V – **R**educed (compression injury)

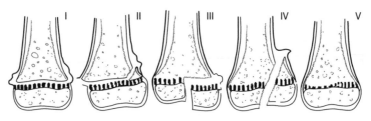

Features of Horner's syndrome

SPAM

Sunken eyeballs (enophthalmos)/**S**ympathetic plexus (cervical) affected
Ptosis
Anhidrosis
Meiosis

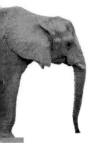

6. Orthopaedics

General

Causes of acute single joint pathology

SINGLe JOINT

Septic arthritis
Internal derangement (eg meniscal tear)
Neuropathic (Charcot's)
Gout (and pseudogout)
Lyme disease
Juvenile or adult rheumatoid arthritis
Osteoarthritis
Ischaemia (avascular necrosis)
Neoplasm, eg pigmented villonodular synovitis
Trauma

X-ray features of osteoarthritis

LOSS

Loss of joint space
Osteophytes (marginal and central)
Subchondral sclerosis
Subchondral cysts

Causes of arthritis with demineralisation

HORSE

Haemophilia
Osteomyelitis
Rheumatoid arthritis
Reiter's disease
Scleroderma
Erythematosus (systemic lupus)

Causes of premature osteoarthritis

COME CHAT

Calcium pyrophosphate dihydrate arthropathy
Ochronosis
Marfan's syndrome
Epiphyseal dysplasia
Charcot arthropathy
Haemophilic arthropathy
Acromegaly
Trauma

Radiological features of rheumatoid arthritis

LESS

Loss of joint space
Erosions
Soft tissue swelling
Soft bones (osteopenia)

Diagnostic criteria for rheumatoid arthritis

MARS

≥ 4 or more of seven for $>6/52$:
Morning stiffness >1 h
Arthritis ≥ 3 joints / **A**rthritis of hand joints (wrist, MCPJ or PIPJ)

Rheumatoid nodules/**R**heumatoid factor/**R**adiological changes, ie LESS (see above)
Symmetrical arthritis

Cardinal features of rheumatoid arthritis

RHEUMATOID

Rheumatoid factor (anti-IgG)
HLA-DR4/**H**LA-Dw4
ESR increase/**E**xtra-articular features (eg restrictive lung disease)
Ulnar deviation
Morning stiffness/**M**etacarpophalangeal joint subluxation
Ankylosis/**A**tlantoaxial joint subluxation/**A**utoimmune/**A**ntinuclear antibody positive
T-cells (CD4)
Osteopaenia
Inflammatory synovial tissue (pannus)
Deformities (eg swan-neck, boutonniere)

Features of Reiter's disease

Can't see, can't pee, and can't bend the knee

Triad of features:
Conjuctivitis (can't see)
Urethritis (can't pee)
Arthritis (can't bend the knee)

Causes of Charcot arthropathy

DS6

Diabetes
Syphilis
Steroids
Spinal cord injury
Spina bifida
Syringomyelia
Scleroderma

Radiological features of Charcot arthropathy
5Ds

Dense subchondral bone
Destruction of articular cortex
Deformity (pencil point)
Debris (loose bodies)
Dislocation

Features of osteomalacia
Vitamin D deficiency in ADULT

Acetabuli protrusio
Decreased bone density
Under-mineralisation of osteoid
Looser's zones (pseudofracture)
Triradiate pelvis (in females)

Causes of pseudofractures
POOF

Paget's disease
Osteomalacia
Osteogenesis imperfecta
Fibrous dysplasia

Features of Paget's disease
ABCD P2M2

Arthritis
Blood flow increase
Cranial nerve compression
Deformity
Pain
Pseudoarthrosis
Metabolic complications
Malignant transformation

Phases of Paget's disease

LAB

Lytic phase: a 'front' of osteoclastic resorption is seen, usually near metaphyseal region of a long bone or osteoporosis circumscripta in the skull
Active phase: both osteoclastic resorption and osteoblastic bone formation occur in the same area of bone
'**B**urnt out' phase: a dense mosaic pattern of bone is seen with little cellular activity

Features of tuberculosis

4 Cs

Caseation
Calcification
Cavitation
Cicatrisation

Causes of chondrocalcinosis

WHIP A DOG

Wilson's disease
Hyperparathyroidism/**H**yperthyroidism/**H**aemochromatosis/**H**aemophilia
Idiopathic (ageing)
Pseudogout
Amyloid/**A**rthritis (rheumatoid, osteoarthritis)
Diabetes mellitus
Ochronosis
Gout

Medical treatment of tuberculosis

RIPES

Rifampicin
Isoniazid
Pyrazinamide
Ethambutol
Streptomycin

Tumours

Tumours that commonly metastasise to bone

Particular Tumours Love Killing Bone

Prostate
Thyroid
Lung
Kidney
Breast

Blastic metastases

5 Bs Lick Pollen

Brain (medulloblastoma)
Bronchus
Breast
Bowel
Bladder
Lymphoma
Prostate

Calcifying metastases

BOTTOM

Breast
Osteosarcoma
Testicular

Thyroid
Ovary
Mucinous cystadenocarcinoma of the GI tract

Differential diagnosis of sclerotic bone lesions

VINDICATE

Vascular, eg haemangioma
Infection, eg osteomyelitis
Neoplasm, eg metastasis
Drugs, eg fluoride
Idiopathic
Congenital, eg osteopetrosis
Autoimmune
Trauma
Endocrine, eg hyperparathyroidism

Differential diagnosis of solitary lucent bone lesions

FOG MACHINES

Fibrous dysplasia
Osteoblastoma
Giant cell tumour
Metastasis
Myeloma
Aneurysmal bone cyst
Chondroblastoma
Chondromyxoid fibroma
Hyperparathyroidism (brown tumours)
Haemangioma
Infection
Non-ossifying fibroma
Eosinophilic granuloma
Enchondroma
Simple/solitary bone cyst

Differential diagnosis of moth-eaten bone destruction

H LEMMON

Histiocytosis X
Lymphoma
Ewing's sarcoma
Metastasis
Multiple myeloma
Osteomyelitis
Neuroblastoma

Sarcomas by age

Every Other Runner Feels Crampy Pain On Moving

Ewing's sarcoma	0–10
Osteosarcoma	10–30
Reticulum cell sarcoma	20–40
Fibrosarcoma	20–40
Chondrosarcoma	40–50
Parosteal sarcoma	40–50
Osteosarcoma	60–70
Metastases	60–70

Features of osteosarcoma

PEARL HARBOR

Paget's disease (10–20%)[*]
Early age (10–20 years)
Around the knee
Raised periosteum by expanding tumour = **sunburst pattern** (similar pattern to Japanese Navy emblem during World War II)
Lace-like architecture
Hyaline arteriosclerosis
Alkaline phosphatase increased
Retinoblastoma[*]

Boys predominantly affected
Osteomyelitis is a differential
Radiation*
*Indicates predisposing factors

Lesions commonly found at apophyses

CAGI

Chondroblastoma
Aneurysmal bone cyst
Giant cell tumour
Infection

Differential diagnosis of round cell tumours

LEMON

Leukaemia/**L**ymphoma
Ewing's sarcoma/**E**osinophilic granuloma
Multiple myeloma
Osteomyelitis
Neuroblastoma

Lesions commonly found at epiphyses

DELCCO

Degenerative
Enchondroma
Lipoma
Cyst
Chondroblastoma
Osteomyelitis

Upper limb

Stages of frozen shoulder

Freezing, Frozen, Thawing

> **Freezing** (inflammatory stage)
> **Frozen** (stiffening due to scarring)
> **Thawing** (resolution)

Types of shoulder instability

TUBS and AMBRI

> **T**raumatic mechanism
> **U**nidirectional and **U**nilateral
> **B**ankart lesion seen
> **S**urgery often required
> **A**traumatic mechanism
> **M**ultidirectional instability
> **B**ilateral shoulder involvement
> **R**ehabilitation needed
> **I**nferior capsular shift surgery

Destruction of medial end of clavicle on X-rays

MILERS

> **M**etastases
> **I**nfection
> **L**ymphoma
> **E**osinophilic granuloma
> **R**heumatoid arthritis
> **S**arcoma

Hand deformities in nerve palsies

DR CUMA

Drop wrist   **R**adial nerve
Claw hand   **U**lnar nerve
Median nerve   **A**pe hand

Causes of median nerve entrapment

MEDIAN TRAP

Myxoedema (hypothyroidism)
o**E**dema (eg premenstrual)
Diabetes
Idiopathic (most common)
Acromegaly
Neoplasm
Trauma
Rheumatoid arthritis
Amyloidosis
Pregnancy

Dupuytren's diathesis

BEG MY Family

Bilateral
Ectopic disease (eg Ledderhose's)
Garrod's knuckle pads
Male
Young
Family history

Dupuytren's contracture: associations

DEAFEST PAIL

Diabetes mellitus
Epilepsy
Age (positive correlation)
Family history (autosomal dominant)/**F**ibromatoses,
eg Ledderhose's
Epileptic medication (eg phenobarbitone)
Smoking
Trauma and heavy manual labour
Peyronie's disease
AIDS
Idiopathic (most common)
Liver disease (secondary to alcohol)

Ray involvement in syndactyly

5:15:50:30

5%   Thumb to index
15%   Index to middle
50%   Middle to ring
30%   Ring to little

Differential diagnosis of lucent lesion in the phalanges on X-rays

GAMES PAGES

Glomus tumour
Arthritis (gout, rheumatoid)
Metastasis (lung, breast)
Enchondroma
Solitary bone cyst
Pancreatitis
Aneurysmal bone cyst
Giant cell tumour
Epidermoid inclusion cyst
Sarcoid

Spine and lower limb

Causes of back pain

DISK MASS

Degeneration
Infection: pelvic inflammatory disease, TB, osteomyelitis/**I**njury (fracture)
Spondylitis, eg spondyloarthropathies such as ankylosing spondylitis
Kidney, eg stones, infection
Multiple **m**yeloma; **M**etastasis from breast, prostate, lung, thyroid and kidney carcinoma
Aneurysm: abdominal pain referred to the back
Slipped disk
Spondylolisthesis

Extra-articular manifestations of ankylosing spondylitis

6 As

Atlanto-axial subluxation
Anterior uveitis
Apical lung fibrosis
Aortic incompetence
Amyloidosis
Autoimmune bowel disease

Features of Scheuermann's disease

All the Ss

Skeletally immature adolescents
Strong hereditary tendency
Sorensen's criteria for diagnosis
    Thoracic kyphosis >45°
    Wedging >5° of 3 adjacent vertebrae
    Thoracolumbar kyphosis >30°
Associated with
    Spondylolysis
    Scoliosis
Schmorl's nodes on X-rays

Waddell's inappropriate signs for back pain

NO CRAP

Non-anatomic tenderness to light touch/**N**on-dermatomal sensory loss
Overreaction, eg disproportionate facial expressions
Cogwheel (give-way) weakness
Raising straight leg (discrepancy between findings on sitting and supine straight leg raising tests)
Axial compression causes pain (vertical loading on a standing patient's skull produces low back pain)
Pelvic rotation causes pain

Evaluation of vertebral fractures to determine underlying cause

Screen for TOMEO

Tumours (X-ray, bone scan, CT)
Osteopaenia (DEXA scan)
Marrow disease (FBC, electrophoresis)
Endocrine disease (thyroid, diabetes, cortisol)
Osteomalacia

Causes of vertebra plana

The vertebral body MELTS away

Myeloma/**M**etastasis
Eosinophilic granuloma
Lymphoma
Trauma/**T**uberculosis
SAPHO syndrome (**S**ynovitis, **A**cne, **P**ustulosis,
Hyperostosis and **O**steitis)

Causes of protrusio acetabuli

All the Os

Osteoporosis
Osteomalacia
Osteogenesis imperfecta
Oh no, not rheumatoid!
Osteoarthritis
Otto pelvis
Rickets, eg X-linked hyp**O**phosphataemic rickets

Paediatric orthopaedics

When to be concerned in paediatric orthopaedics

When children present with the 5 Ss

Symptoms
Stiffness
a**S**ymmetry
Syndromes
Systemic disorders

Common causes of a limp in children (by age)

The limping child DIPS

Age	Condition
Birth	**D**DH
0–5	**I**nfection
5–10	**P**erthes' disease
10–15	**S**CFE

Incidence of some paediatric conditions

1 in 1000, 10,000 and 100,000

1/1000	DDH/CTEV/metatarsus adductus
1/10,000	Perthes' disease
1/100,000	SCFE

Risk factors for DDH

All the Fs
Female
First-born
Le**F**t side affected
Fluid defect (oligohydramnios)
Faulty position (breech)
Fat (large child)
Female hormones (eg relaxin)

Clinical tests for DDH

dislocataBle and Out to in

Barlow's test	Is the hip dislocata**B**le?
Ortolani's test	Is the hip reducible? (from **O**ut to in)

Diagnostic criteria for Still's disease (systemic onset juvenile idiopathic arthritis)

IF I had passed the MRCGP

Intermittent **F**ever (high with 2 daily spikes up to 40°C)
Iridocyclitis
Maculopapular salmon pink rash
Rheumatoid factor positive
Cervical spine involvement
Generalised lymphadenopathy and hepatosplenomegaly
Pericarditis

Clinical features of sickle cell disease

HBSS PAIN CRISIS

Haemolysis/***H**and–foot syndrome (dactylitis)*
***B**one marrow hyperplasia*
***S**troke (thrombotic or haemorrhagic)*, **S**ubarachnoid bleeding
***S**kin ulcers (usually leg)*
***P**ain crises*/**P**riapism/**P**sychosocial problems
Anaemia/**A**plastic crisis/***A**vascular necrosis*
***I**nfections (bone, joint, CNS, pulmonary, genitourinary)*
Nocturia (urinary frequency)
Cholelithiasis/**C**ardiomegaly/**C**ongestive heart failure/**C**hest syndrome
Retinopathy/**R**enal failure/**R**enal concentration defects
***I**nfarction (bone, muscle, spleen, bowel, renal, CNS)*
Sequestration crisis (spleen, liver)
Increased foetal loss in pregnancy
***S**epsis*
(Problems relevant to orthopaedics in italics)

Diagnostic criteria for neurofibromatosis

CAFE SPOT

Cafe-au-lait spots
Axillary or inguinal freckling (Crowe's sign)
Fibroma (neuro)
Eye: Lisch nodules
Skeletal involvement (eg bowing)
Positive family history
Optic **T**umour (glioma)

Duchenne's versus Becker's muscular dystrophy

DMD vs BMD

Duchenne's	**D**oesn't **M**ake **D**ystrophin
Becker's	**B**adly **M**ade **D**ystrophin

Features of trisomy 21 (Down's syndrome)

My CHILD HAS PROBLEM

*M*etatarsus primus varus
Congenital heart disease/**C**ataracts
Hypotonia/**H**ypothyroidism
*I*ncurved little finger
*L*igamentous laxity
Duodenal atresia/**D**elayed development/**D**iabetes
Hirschsprung's disease/*Hip dislocation*
Alzheimer's disease/*Atlantoaxial instability*
Scoliosis/Spondylolisthesis/SCFE
*Patella dislocation/Planovalgus feet/P*rotruding
tongue/**P**almar crease (single)
Round face/**R**olling eye (nystagmus)
Occiput flat/**O**blique eye fissure
Brushfield spot/**B**rachycephaly
Low nasal bridge
Epicanthic fold/**E**ar folded
Mental retardation/**M**yoclonus
(Orthopaedic problems are highlighted in italics)

Some common skeletal dysplasias

MACHO MEN OF GOD

Marfan's syndrome
Achondroplasia
Cleidocranial dysostosis
Hypophosphatemic rickets
Osteogenesis imperfecta
Multiple hereditary exostoses
Enchondromatosis (Ollier's)
Neurofibromatosis
Osteopetrosis
Fibrous dysplasia
Gaucher's disease
Osteopoikilosis
Dactyly, eg syndactyly

Features of Marfan's syndrome

MARFANS

Mitral valve prolapse
Autosomal dominant/**A**rched palate (high)/**A**ortic aneurysm/**A**ortic regurgitation/**A**cetabular protrusion
Retinal detachment and superior dislocation of the lens
Fibrillin mutation on chromosome **F**ifteen
Arachnodactyly
Negative nitroprusside test (differentiates Marfan's from homocystinuria)
Scoliosis/**S**pondylolisthesis/**S**lack joints (ligamentous laxity)/**S**pontaneous pneumothorax/**S**triae atrophicae (stretch marks)

Features of osteopetrosis (marble bone disease)

MARBLES

Multiple fractures
Anaemia
Restricted cranial nerves
Blind and deaf
Liver enlarged
Erlenmeyer flask deformity
Splenomegaly
NB Eponymous name: **Albers**-Schonberg disease =
M**arbles** anagram)

Features of Hurler's syndrome

HURLERS

Hepatosplenomegaly
Ugly facies
Recessive inheritance (autosomal)
L-iduronidase deficiency (alpha)
Eyes (cornea) clouded
Retardation (mental)
Short (**S**tubby) fingers

Causes of frayed metaphyseal appearance on X-rays

CHARMS

Congenital infections (rubella, syphilis)
Hypophosphatasia
Achondroplasia
Rickets
Metaphyseal dysostosis
Scurvy

Causes of Erlenmeyer flask deformity on X-rays

DAMN FROG

Down's syndrome
Achondroplasia
Metaphyseal dysplasia
Niemann–Pick disease
Fibrous dysplasia
Rickets
Osteopetrosis
Gaucher's disease

Causes of transverse lucent metaphyseal lines on X-rays

LINING

Leukaemia
Illness, systemic (rickets, scurvy)
Normal variant
Infection (transplacental – congenital syphilis)
Neuroblastoma metastases
Growth lines

Genetic conditions with blue sclera

MIXED

Marfan's syndrome
Imperfecta (osteogenesis)
Pseudo**X**anthoma Elasticum
Ehlers–**D**anlos syndrome

Causes of Wormian bones on X-rays

PORK CHOPS

Pyknodysostosis
Osteogenesis imperfecta
Rickets (in healing phase)
Kinky hair syndrome (Menke's)
Cleidocranial dysostosis
Hypothyroidism/**H**ypophosphatasia
Otopalatodigital syndrome
Primary acro-osteolysis
Syndrome of Down

Causes of dense sclerotic lines on X-rays

DENSE LINES

D-vitamin intoxication
Elemental arsenic and bismuth
Normal variant
Systemic illness
o**E**strogen to mother during pregnancy
Leukaemia/**L**ead poisoning
Infection (TORCH)/**I**diopathic hypercalcaemia
Never forget rickets
Early hypothyroidism
Scurvy/**S**ickle cell disease

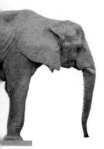

7. Miscellaneous

Types of malignant melanoma

Melanoma Always Spreads to Nodes

(in order of worsening prognosis)
Lentiginous **M**aligna
Acral lentiginous
Superficial spreading
Nodular

Clinical risk factors for malignant melanoma

ABCDE

Asymmetry
Border irregularity
Colour variegation (varying colours)
Diameter (>6 mm is characteristic)
Evolving (ongoing changes)

Clarke's levels for prognosis of malignant melanoma

Freckles Require Judicious Pathological Evaluation

(from deep to superficial, with deep having poorer prognosis)
Fat (level V; worst prognosis: 75% chance of recurrence at 5 years)
Reticular dermis (level IV)
Junction of reticular and papillary dermis (level III)
Papillary dermis (level II)
Epidermis (level I; best prognosis)

Taking a history of breast pathology

LMNOP

Lump (ask about all the features of the lump)
Mammary changes
Nipple discharge/changes
Obvious risk factors, eg previous breast cancer
Pain

Signs of nipple pathology

The 7 Ds

Discoloration
Discharge
Depression (retraction or inversion)
Deviation
Displacement
Destruction
Duplication

Causes of cervical lymphadenopathy

LIST

Lymphoma/**L**eukaemia
Infection
Sarcoidosis
Tumours/**T**uberculosis

Indications for thyroid surgery

The 4 Cs

Cosmesis
Compression (of trachea and/or oesophagus)
Control (of toxic symptoms in hyperthyroidism)
Carcinoma

Complications of thyroid surgery

All the Hs

Immediate:
Haemorrhage, leading to airway obstruction from secondary laryngeal oedema
Hoarseness (damaged recurrent laryngeal nerve)
Hyperthyroidism (known as thyroid storm)

Early:
(**H**)infection (a rather weak H!)
Hypoparathyroidism, leading to **H**ypocalcaemia

Late:
Hyperthyroidism (recurrent)
Hypothyroidism
Hypertrophic scarring

Classification of thyroid eye disease

NO SPECS

Class 0	**N**	**N**o signs or symptoms
Class 1	**O**	**O**nly signs of upper lid retraction and stare, with or without lid lag and exophthalmos
Class 2	**S**	**S**oft tissue involvement
Class 3	**P**	**P**roptosis
Class 4	**E**	**E**xophthalmos
Class 5	**C**	**C**orneal involvement
Class 6	**S**	**S**ight loss due to optic nerve involvement

Risk factors for thyroid cancer

CRISP

Chronic lymphocytic thyroiditis (Hashimoto's disease, which is a risk factor for lymphoma)
Relatives with thyroid cancer (genetics)
Ionising radiation
Solitary thyroid nodule
Prolonged stimulation by raised TSH

Route of spread of thyroid cancer

The last letter rule

Papillar**Y** ends in **Y** = **y**ellow = lymph = lymphatic spread
Follicula**R** ends in **R** = **r**ed = blood = spreads via
bloodstream

Signs of peritonsillar abscess

MOST FIT

Muffled voice
Odynophagia
Swelling
Trismus
Foetid odour
Inflammation
Temperature rise

Phaeochromocytoma

The rule of 10s

10% malignant
10% bilateral
10% in children
10% multiple tumours
10% extra-adrenal (thorax, neck, bladder, kidney, scrotum)
10% familial (von Hippel–Lindau syndrome, MEN I & II)

MEN I (Werner's syndrome)

Type I = Primary = pathology beginning with P

Parathyroid hyperplasia
Pancreatic islet cell tumour:
    Zollinger–Ellison syndrome (50%)
    Insulinoma (20%)
Pituitary tumours

MEN IIA (Sipple's syndrome)

Type 2 = Secondary = Sipple's; patients with MEN IIA drive at 2MPH

Medullary thyroid carcinoma
Phaeochromocytoma
Hyperparathyroidism (parathyroid hyperplasia)

MEN IIB

Patients with MEN IIB enjoy M&Ms in the afternoon (PM)

Medullary thyroid carcinoma
Mucosal neuromas
Phaeochromocytoma
Marfanoid body habitus

Causes of a red eye

GO SUCK

Glaucoma
Orbital disease
Scleritis
Uveitis
Conjunctivitis
Keratitis

Mnemonic index

1,2 – buckle my shoe 2
1,2 – try to screw 56
1,3,5,7,9,11 15
1 in 1000, 10,000 and 100,000
 74
2 from 1, 2 from 2, 2 from 3 15
second letter rule 19
2 STAR 7
3:1:0:3:5:5 6–7
3,4 – Austin Moore 56
3,4 – kick the door 2
3 As and 4 Hs 35
three Bs bend the elbow 9
3 Ds 47
3 DUCks PECking On GRAss
 18
3 Es 55
3 GOOSE and 1 DUCK 12
3 types of MURG 56
4 Cs (thyroid surgery) 82
4 Cs (tuberculosis) 63
5,6 – pick up sticks 2
5:15:50:30 70
5 As 33
5 Bs Lick Pollen 64
5 Ds 62
5 Ps 2
5 Ss 73
6 As (ankylosing spondylitis) 71
6 As (cartilage) 22
6 As (premedication) 34
6 Fs 40

6 Ps 46
7,8 – shut the gate 2
7 Ds 82
8 Cs 32
90% rule 54

A of A of A 12
ABCD P2M2 62
ABCDE (advanced trauma life
 support) 51
ABCDE (melanoma) 81
ABCDEF 39
ABCS (aortic arch branches) 12
ABCS (X-rays) 31
ACIDE 26
AEIOU (renal dialysis) 37
AEIOU (varicose veins) 47
all the Fs 74
all the Hs 83
all the Os 73
all the Ps 54–5
all the Ss 72
AMPLE 53
AMYLASE 42
Aneurysms May Sometimes
 Cause Terrible Bleeding
 46
APPENDICITIS 43
ARDS 36
As 22
as heard on Star Wars, GO
 C3PO 54

As Shops Opened, Colin
Invested Excitedly 38
Astute Anatomists Share Inside
Secrets About Lungs 14
ATOMIC 52
AVPU 51

BAD CaT 48
BBC 8
BEAT ARDS 36
BEDS 31
BEG MY Family 69
bones, stones, moans and
psychic groans 23
BOTTOM 64–5
BrachioRadialis 9
BREAST 11

C3,4,5 keep the diaphragm alive
2
C5,6,7 raise your arms to
heaven 2
CAFE SPOT 76
CAGI 67
Californians Love Girls in String
Bikinis 3
can't see, can't pee and can't
bend the knee 61
CHAPTER 30
CHARM TIPS 40
CHARMS 78
CHIASMA 41
CHIMP 37
CHIPS 36
Colin, He Doesn't See Girls
Much. That's Obvious,
Stupid 5
COLLAGEN 21
COME CHAT 60
Come Enter the Abdomen 14
count 1 to 4 but staggered 14
CRAMPED 45
CRAMPING 22

CRIMP PRINTS 35
CRISP 83
CRITOL 9–10
Curtis Can't Count Bones, Never
Took Calculus 18

D SCUM 38
DAMN FROG 79
DEAFEST PAIL 70
DELCCO 67
DELIRIUM 33
DENSE LINES 80
DISK MASS 71
dislocataBle and Out to in 74
DMD vs BMD 76
DOPE 24
DR CUMA 69
Dressed In A Surgeon's Gown,
A Physician May Make
Some Initial Temporary
Progress 29
DS6 61

ECCCI 37
Every Other Runner Feels
Crampy Pain On Moving
66

FLEDD 44
FOG MACHINES 65
Freckles Require Judicious
Pathological Evaluation
81
freezing, frozen, thawing 68
FRIEND 45
Friendly Irish Anaesthetist
Offers Ronaldo A Painless
Tendon 16

GA LAW and COUCH 41–2
GAMES PAGES 70
GARDENS 46
GET SMASHED 41

GFR 15
GLASS 3
GO C3PO 54
GO SUCK 85
grade I to III then ABC 54

H LEMMON 66
HASH 34
HBSS PAIN CRISIS 75
HEAVE 47
HEMATURIA 48
HI CALCIUM Produces Stones
    23
HI POTASSIuM 22
HORSE 60
HURLERS 78

I AM SCARED 53
I CHOP 40
I Get Lost On Fridays 15
I Like To Rise So High 13
I WAS HOPPING MAD 25
IATROGENIC 38
IF I had passed the MRCGP 75
Immunodeficiency May Directly
    Cause Life-threatening
    Sepsis 26

LAB 63
LaDy between two MAJORS 8
last letter rule 84
lateral is less, medial is more 7
LEMON 67
LESS 60
LIFELESS 27
like a game of tennis 53
like taking more and more
    cOCAINe 52
limping child DIPS 74
LINING 79
LIST 82
LML 7
LMNOP 82

LOAF 11
LORD help these patients!
    36–7
LOSS 59
Love-15-30-40 53
LR6, SO4 and the rest by 3 4
LSD 6
Luscious Fried Tomatoes Sit
    Naked In Anticipation Of
    Sauce 4

MACHO MEN OF GOD 77
MARBLES 78
MARFANS 77
MARS 60–1
May I Slowly String Cat Gut? 5
MEDIAN TRAP 69
Medical Schools Let Confident
    People In 6
Melanoma Always Spreads to
    Nodes 81
MILERS 68
Miss Mary Makes Me Unhappy
    7
MIXED 79
MOST FIT 84
Muscle Contraction Results
    Mainly Through Sustained
    Action Potentials 27
Muscles Support the Pharynx
    and Larynx 1
My CHILD HAS PROBLEM 76

NAVEL 16
NO CRAP 72
NO SPECS 83
NoaH Told MariaH To Try
    Cervical Counting 4

Only Real Frail Admissions
    Require Care 34
OVALE 3

P-THORAX 52
PAD and DAB 11
PANCREAS (complications of pancreatitis) 42–3
PANCREAS (treatment of pancreatitis) 42
Particular Tumours Love Killing Bone 64
patients with MEN IIA drive at 2MPH 85
patients with MEN IIB enjoy M&Ms in the afternoon 85
PEARL HARBOR 66–7
Piles Don't Contribute To A Good Sex Life 16
PLASTIC RAG 24–5
Players Follow Pimps For Fun 10
Point and Shoot 16
POOF 62
PORK CHOPS 80
Pretty Girls Often Get Old Quickly 17
PRICE 51
PRO AND CON 32
Put My Leg Down Please 18
PVT LEFT BATTLE 12

Really Need Booze To Be At My Nicest 9
RHEUMATOID 61
ride a LONG way on the SUPRAhighway 8
RIPES 64
Robert Taylor Drinks Cold Beer 6
rule of 2s 44
rule of 3s 39
rule of 10s 84

S2,3,4 keep the erection, urine and faeces off the floor 2

SAD PUCKER 13
SALT 6
SALTED 23
SALTR 56
SAPHO 73
Say Grace before Tea 18
SCALP 3
SCOPE 35
screen for TOMEO 72
second letter rule 19
Send The Lord To Say A Prayer 8
SHIP 32
Should The Children Ever Find Lumps Readily 30
SINGLe JOINT 59
SITS 7
So May I Always Love Sally 17
SOCRATES 30
Some Anatomists Like Fishfingers, Others Prefer Sausage & Mash 5
Some Damn Englishman Called It The Testis 17
Some Lovers Try Positions That They Cannot Handle 10
Some Tend To Nicely Stop Clots 24
Sometimes Intestines Get Really Stretched Causing Leakage 13
SPAM 57
SPLINT 55
STOMA BAGS HELP 44–5

TEAM 55
TESTIS 49
THE THEATRES 48–9
TIN CAN BED 31
Tom, Dick and A Very Nervous Harry 19
Tom Has A Very Nasty Dirty Pill 19

TOM SCHREPFER 33
TUBS and AMBRI 68
type 1 = Primary = pathology
     beginning with P 84
type 2 = Secondary = Sipple's
     85

VEM 52
vertebral body MELTS away 73
VINDICATE 65
VIRchow 24

vitamin D deficiency in ADULT
     62
VITAMINS A, B, C, D, E 25–6

walk a SHORT way to the street
     CORner 8
WBC 47
when children present with the
     5 Ss 73
WHIP A DOG 63
WRAP IF HOT 43

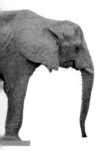

Subject index

abdominal aorta 13
abdominal pain 43
adrenal cortex 15
adult respiratory distress
        syndrome (ARDS)
    causes 36
    management 36
advanced trauma life support
        (ATLS)
    definition 51
    disability assessment 51
    Glasgow coma score 52
    primary survey 52
Albers–Schönberg disease 78
allergy 26
amputation 47
amylase, raised 42
anaemia, sickle cell 75
anaesthesia
    aims 33
    premedication 34
aneurysm 46
ankle
    eversion/inversion 19
    structures passing behind
        medial malleolus 19
    structures passing in front of
        ankle 19
ankylosing spondylitis 71
antibiotics for tuberculosis 64
anticoagulants 24
aortic branches

abdominal 13
arch 12
aortic hiatus 14
apophyseal lesions 67
apoptosis 27
appendicitis 43
ARDS (adult respiratory distress
        syndrome)
    causes 36
    management 36
arm see upper limb
arthritis
    ankylosing spondylitis 71
    demineralisation and 60
    osteoarthritis 59, 60
    Reiter's disease 61
    rheumatoid 60–1
    Still's disease 75
arthroplasty 56
ATLS see advanced trauma life
        support
audit 38
avascular necrosis 24–5
axillary artery 8

back pain
    diagnosis 71
    Waddell's inappropriate signs
        72
Becker's muscular dystrophy 76
biceps, origins of heads 8
bicipital groove 8

biliary tract disease 40
blastic metastases 64
blood gases, hypoxia 34–5
blood loss, in trauma 53
bone
  apophyseal lesions 67
  dysplasia 77
  epiphyseal lesions 67
  Erlenmeyer flask deformity 79
  fracture *see* fracture
  lucent lesions 65, 70, 79
  metaphyseal lesions 78, 79
  metastases 64
  moth-eaten lesions 66
  osteomalacia 62
  osteopetrosis 78
  osteosarcoma 66–7
  Paget's disease 62–3
  pseudofracture 62
  round cell tumours 67
  sclerotic lesions 65
  sclerotic lines 80
  Wormian bones 80
brachial plexus 6–7
brachioradialis muscle 9
branchial arches 1
breast pathology
  nipples 82
  taking a history 82

calcification
  cartilage 63
  metastases 64–5
calcium, high
  causes 23
  symptoms 23
cancer *see* tumours
cardiac muscle 27
carotid artery 5
carpal bones 10
cartilage 22
  chondrocalcinosis 63

catheters 36
caval foramen 14
central line insertion 36
cervical lymphadenopathy 82
cervical nerves 2
cervical vertebrae 4
Charcot arthropathy
  causes 61
  X-rays 62
cholelithiasis 40
chondrocalcinosis 63
Clarke's levels (prognosis of
  melanoma) 81
clavicle 68
clinical audit 38
clinical examination
  cutaneous ulcers 31
  lumps 30
coagulation, warfarin and 24
collagen 21
compartment syndrome 54–5
confusion, postoperative 33
consciousness, assessment
  51–2
consent 32
corticosteroids 25
cranial nerves 4
cubital fossa 9

DDH (developmental dysplasia
  of the hip)
  risk factors 74
  tests for 74
describing a disease 29
developmental dysplasia of the
  hip *see* DDH
diagnosis, general
  clinical examination 30–1
  description of a disease 29
  differential diagnosis 31
  history-taking 30
  X-rays 31

dialysis 37
diaphragm 14
differential diagnosis 31
digits
   lucent lesions 70
   syndactyly 70
disability assessment in ATLS 51
   see also Glasgow coma score
disease, standard description of 29
dislocation
   hip 54, 74
   shoulder 54, 55
Down's syndrome 76
Duchenne's muscular dystrophy 76
duodenal anatomy 14
duodenal ulcer 40
Dupuytren's contracture 70
Dupuytren's diathesis 69

elbow
   brachioradialis muscle 9
   cubital fossa contents 9
   flexors 9
   ossification centres 9–10
embolism, pulmonary 33
epidemiology
   paediatric conditions 74
   screening programmes 38
   study designs 37
epiphyseal lesions 67
Erlenmeyer flask deformity 79
examination
   cutaneous ulcers 31
   lumps 30
external carotid artery 5
extraocular muscles, nerves supplying 4
eye
   blue sclera 79
   red eye 85
   thyroid disease 83

femoral artery 18
femoral sheath 16
femoral triangle 17
femur
   external rotators 17
   fracture 56
fever, postoperative 32
fingers
   lucent lesions 70
   syndactyly 70
fistula, prevention of closure 45
foot 18
foramen ovale 3
forearm
   fracture 56
   muscles 10
fracture
   classification (general) 54
   classification of fractures around the physis 56
   classification of open fractures 54
   delayed union 55
   hip 56
   spine 72
   upper limb 56
frozen shoulder 68

Galeazzi fracture 56
gallstones 40
Gardner's syndrome 46
gargoylism 78
gastric ulcer 40
gastrointestinal tract
   appendicitis 43
   duodenal anatomy 14
   fistulae 45
   functional obstruction 45
   Gardner's syndrome 46

gastrointestinal tract (continued)
  Meckel's diverticulum 44
  oesophageal cancer 39
  peptic ulcer 40
  stomas 44–5
genitourinary tract, male
  penis 16
  scrotal layers 17
  scrotal swelling 48–9
  spermatic cord 16
  undescended testis 49
Glasgow coma score 52
glossopharnygeus muscle 1
Gustillo–Anderson classification
      of open fractures 54

haematuria 48
haemorrhage, in trauma 53
hand
  Dupuytren's disease 69–70
  muscles 11–12
  nerve palsies 69
  phalangeal lesions 70
  syndactyly 70
head, anatomy 3–4
healing, delayed
  fractures 55
  wounds 25–6
heart muscle 27
hepatomegaly 40
hernia, umbilical 39
hip
  DDH 74
  dislocation 54, 74
  fracture 56
  protrusio acetabuli 73
  rotator muscles 17
history-taking
  breast pathology 82
  pain 30
  social situation 30
  trauma cases 53

Horner's syndrome 57
humerus, muscles attached to 8
Hurler's syndrome 78
hyoid arch 1
hyoid bone, muscles attached to
  5
hypercalcaemia
  causes 23
  symptoms 23
hyperkalaemia 22
hypernatraemia 23
hypersensitivity 26
hypokalaemia 22
hypoxia
  patients at risk 35
  types and causes 34

iliac fossa, pain in 43
immune disorders
  acquired immunodeficiency
    26
  hypersensitivity 26
incidence, paediatric conditions
  74
inferior vena cava 13
inguinal canal 16
intensive care, transfer to 34
internal jugular vein 6
interossei muscles 11
intubation 35
ischaemia
  acute limb 46
  avascular necrosis 24–5

joints
  arthritis 59–61, 75
  causes of single joint
      pathology 59
  Charcot arthropathy 61–2
  dislocation 54, 55, 74
jugular vein 6
juvenile idiopathic arthritis 75

kidney failure *see* renal failure
Kocher's manoeuvre 55

larynx 1
leg *see* hip; lower limb
limps, in children 74
liver, hepatomegaly 40
lower limb
  acute ischaemia 46
  amputation 47
  anatomy 17–19
  see also hip
lumbar plexus
  branches 15
  roots 15
lumps
  clinical examination 30
  scrotal swellings 48–9
lung
  bronchopulmonary segments
    14
  pneumothorax 52
lymphadenopathy 82

malleolus, medial, structures
    passing behind 19
mandibular arch 1
marble bone disease 78
Marfan's syndrome 77
mechanical ventilation 35
Meckel's cartilage 1
Meckel's diverticulum 44
median nerve
  comparison with ulnar nerve
    11
  entrapment 69
  supplying the hand 11
mediastinal anatomy
  posterior 12
  superior 12
melanoma
  prognosis 81

risk factors 81
  types 81
MEN *see* multiple endocrine
    neoplasia
metaphyses
  frayed appearance 78
  lucent lines 79
metastasis
  blastic 64
  calcifying 64–5
  tumours commonly
    metastasing to bone 64
Monteggia fracture 56
multiple endocrine neoplasia
    (MEN)
  type I 84
  type IIA 85
  type IIB 85
muscles
  anatomy of the head & neck 5
  anatomy of the lower limb
    17–18
  anatomy of the upper limb
    7–8, 9, 10, 11, 12
  potentially absent 2
  tissue types 27
  see also soft tissue injury
muscular dystrophy 76
musculocutaneous nerve 8

naevus 81
neck *see* cervical *entries*
necrosis
  avascular 24–5
  compared to apoptosis 27
nerves
  lumbar plexus 15
  passing through supraorbital
    fissure 4
  reflex roots 2
  supplying the extraocular
    muscles 4

nerves (continued)
  supplying the scalp 3
  supplying the trunk 2
  supplying the upper limb 2,
    6–7, 8, 11
  upper limb neuropathy 69
neurofibromatosis 76
neuropathic joints 61–2
nipple pathology 82

obstruction, GI tract 45
oesophageal cancer 39
oesophageal hiatus 14
osteitis deformans *see* Paget's
    disease
osteoarthritis
  premature 60
  X-rays 59
osteomalacia 62
osteopetrosis 78
osteosarcoma 66–7
Otto's disease (protrusio
    acetabuli) 73
oxygen *see* hypoxia

paediatrics
  elbow ossification 9–10
  epidemiology 74
  limping 74
  orthopaedic conditions 74–80
  orthopaedic danger signs 73
  umbilical hernia 39
Paget's disease of bone
  features 62
  phases 63
pain
  in the back 71, 72
  in right iliac fossa 43
  taking a history 30
pancreatitis
  causes 41
  complications 42–3
  prognosis 41–2

raised amylase 42
  treatment 42
pectoralis muscles, nerves
    supplying 7
penis 16
peptic ulcer 40
peritonsillar abscess 84
pes anserinus 18
phaeochromocytoma 84
phalanges 70
pharyngeal arches 1
phrenic nerve 2
pneumothorax 52
polyposis, Gardner's syndrome
    46
postoperative conditions
  common complications 32
  confusion 33
  pyrexia 32
potassium
  high 22
  low 22
premedication 34
primary survey 52
procollagen 21
protrusio acetabuli 73
pseudofracture 62
pulmonary embolism 33
pyrexia, postoperative 32

radial nerve 11
radiography
  Charcot arthropathy 62
  interpretation 31
  osteoarthritis 59
  rheumatoid arthritis 60
Ranson's criteria (pancreatitis)
    41–2
Raynaud's phenomenon
  causes 48
  skin changes 47
reactive arthritis *see* Reiter's
    disease

red eye 85
reflex roots 2
Reiter's disease 61
renal failure
    indications for dialysis 37
    patients at risk 36–7
    renal causes 37
respiratory system
    disorders 35–6
    lung anatomy 14
    pneumothorax 52
retroperitoneal structures 13
rheumatoid arthritis
    diagnosis 60–1
    features of 61
    X-rays 60
road traffic accidents 53
rotator cuff, muscles 7
round cell tumours 67

sacral nerves 2
Salter–Harris classification of
        fractures 56
sarcoma
    incidence by age 66
    osteosarcoma 66–7
scalp
    layers 3
    nerves supplying 3
scapula 8
sclera, blue 79
screening programmes
    criteria for 38
    problems with 38
scrotal layers 17
scrotal swelling 48–9
serratus anterior muscle, nerves
        supplying 2, 6
Sheuermann's disease 72
shoulder
    attachment of biceps 8
    dislocation, anterior 54, 55
    dislocation, posterior 55

frozen 68
    instability of 68
    rotator cuff 7
sickle cell disease 75
Sipple's syndrome 85
skeletal dysplasia 77
skeletal muscle 27
skin
    layers 3
    ulcers 31
smooth muscle 27
social history-taking 30
sodium, high 23
soft tissue injury
    compartment syndrome 54–5
    general management 51
    wound healing 25–6
spermatic cord 16
spine
    cervical vertebrae 4
    fracture 72
    Sheuermann's disease 72
    vertebra plana 73
    see also back pain
spleen
    anatomy 15
    splenomegaly 41
sternoclavicular joint 68
steroids 25
Still's disease 75
stoma
    complications of 44–5
    indications for 44
stomach ulcer 40
study designs 37
stylopharnygeus muscle 1
supraorbital fissure 4
sutural (Wormian) bones 80
syndactyly 70

tarsal bones 18
tendons, pes anserinus 18
testis, undescended 49

thigh, medial compartment 18
thoracic nerve of Bell 2
thrombosis
  prognosis 24
  risk factors 24
thyroid artery 5
thyroid cancer
  risk factors 83
  spread 84
thyroid eye disease 83
thyroid surgery
  complications 83
  indications 82
tonsils 84
tracheostomy 35
trisomy 21 76
tuberculosis
  features 63
  treatment 64
tumours
  breast 82
  melanoma 81
  MEN 84–5
  metastases 64–5
  oesophagus 39
  phaeochromocytoma 84
  round cell 67
  sarcoma 66–7
  thyroid 83–4

ulcer
  cutaneous 31
  peptic 40
ulnar nerve
  comparison with median
    nerve 11
  supplying interossei muscles
    11
umbilical hernia 39
upper limb
  acute ischaemia 46
  amputation 47

anatomy 6–12
fracture 56
see also hand; shoulder
urology
  haematuria 48
  see also genitourinary tract,
    male

varicose veins 47
vascular system
  anatomy 5–6, 8, 12–13, 18
  conditions requiring surgery
    46–8
  thrombosis & embolism 24,
    33
vena cava 13
venous insufficiency 47
venous thrombosis
  prognosis 24
  risk factors 24
ventilation, assisted 35
vertebra plana 73
vertebral column *see* spine
Virchow's triad 24
volar superficial group of
  muscles 10

Waddell's inappropriate signs for
  back pain 72
warfarin 24
webbing of fingers 70
Wermer's syndrome 84
Wormian bones 80
wound healing 25–6
wrist 10

X-rays
  Charcot arthropathy 62
  interpretation 31
  osteoarthritis 59
  rheumatoid arthritis 60